TO FIND THE CAUSES OF STRESS IN LADY DOCTORS OF PUBLIC AND PRIVATE HOSPITALS IN PESHAWAR DISTRICT

KHYBER MEDICAL COLLEGE

PESHAWAR

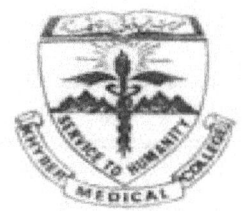

TABLE OF CONTENTS

APPROVAL SHEET

This is to certify that project titled **"To find the causes of stress in lady doctors of Public and Private hospitals in Peshawar District"** has been successfully completed by students of batch no.5, 4th year MBBS session 2013-14.

Project Director:

Waleed Mabood

Approved by:

Dr. Bushra   _____

Head, Department Of Community Medicine

K.M.C, Peshawar

Supervised by:

Dr. Romana   _____

Assistant Professor

Community Medicine Department

K.M.C, Peshawar

DEPARTMENT OF COMMUNITY MEDICINE

KHYBER MEDICAL COLLEGE PESHAWAR

To the efforts and commitment of all those lady doctors who work day and night to save lives in hospitals along with playing multiple roles in society as a responsible daughter, sister, wife and a mother!

ABSTRACT

Background: Stress has become a public health menace of the day. It cannot be eliminated from life and it's absolutely essential that we learn to manage it. Stress management is of special relevance to female doctors who encounter extreme challenges in their professional and personal life. Diagnosing the type of stressors that they come across and experience assumes greater significance. It will pave the way for working out appropriate coping strategies and interventions. This research presents a review of existing empirical studies and literature on the nature and types of environmental demands and pressures that doctors have to face globally.

These studies have focused on the impairment that stress causes among lady doctors with respect to workload, demands and challenges; problems in interpersonal communication, professional aspirations, burden of administration, environmental hazards, security issues, low salaries, legal threats, suicidal tendencies and family life. Some coping mechanisms for the management of stress and interventions from organizational as well as from the individual points of view to choose a proactive life, focusing on 'positive internalizations' have been suggested at the end.

Aim: To evaluate the causes of stress in lady doctors of government and private hospitals in district Peshawar and to compare and contrast the obtained results in different age groups.

Methods: This was a cross-sectional study that took place in the city of Peshawar. The study was conducted from March 2013-August 2013. The sample age that this research was directed at was from 24-60 years of lady doctors. The group of population that was studied was lady doctors working in government and private hospitals from different specialties of 4 tertiary care hospitals, out of which 2 were government run and 2 privately run. The data collection tool was self-designed questionnaire, consisting of 22 questions. Data about causes of stress was collected by inquiring about workload, working hours, salary, burn out phenomena, family-work conflict and major causes leading to stress.

Results: Workload being the most common stressor was found to be 72% in public sector hospitals while the rate being shockingly low in private hospitals that is about 28%. Low salary, uncooperative patients, hostile environment and non-supporting staff was found to be 70%, 54%, 52%, and 52% while in private sector it was 30%, 46%, 48 % and 48 %, respectively. Burden of administration, exhaustion and lack of time and recognition were variables found at higher rate in private sect. that are 54%, 75% and 61% respectively. Stressors that were found in young doctors from age group 24-30 irrespective of the sector are insecurity, exams and studies stress, vulnerability to diseases, burnt out phenomena, self-criticism, peer pressure and social expectations which rated 56%, 68%, 54%, 54%, 56%, 47% and 55% respectively. Married workgroup stressors were uncooperative husband, burden of children and satisfaction of household chores which are 65%, 37% and 62% in public hospitals while 35%, 63% and 38% in private hospitals, respectively.

Conclusion: According to results, lady doctors of government hospitals were mostly affected by workload, low salaries and hostility faced by them from senior staff. While private hospital lady doctors couldn't cope with the administrative responsibilities, lack of leisure time and recognition. The age group 24-30 was affected massively because of lack of security, risk to acquire diseases, burden of exams, peer pressure and social expectations and obligations while the married group was affected by domestic non-compliance and fulfilling the dual role responsibilities. Some productive measures both at individual and occupation system level needs to be taken such as protection from unhygienic and unproductive occupational stress, offering them equitable salaries, protected time and means of covering small crises at home and at work by flexible hours, freedom to fail and providing open-minded mentors may help reduce the stress factors to significant level.

Keywords: *Lady doctors, District Peshawar, Government sector hospitals, Private sector hospitals, Stress, Young doctors, Married doctors, Workload, Family-work conflict*

INTRODUCTION

Stress

Stress is a normal physical response to events that make you feel threatened or upset your balance in some way. When you sense danger — whether it's real or imagined — the body's defenses kick into high gear in a rapid, automatic process known as the "fight-or-flight" reaction, or the *stress response*.

The stress response is the body's way of protecting you. When working properly, it helps you stay focused, energetic, and alert. In emergency situations, stress can save your life — giving you extra strength to defend yourself, for example, or spurring you to slam on the brakes to avoid an accident.

But beyond a certain point, stress stops being helpful and starts causing major damage to your health, your mood, your productivity, your relationships, and your quality of life[1]

Response to stress

It's important to learn how to recognize when your stress levels are out of control. The most dangerous thing about stress is how easily it can creep up on you. You get used to it. It starts to feels familiar even normal. You don't notice how much it's affecting you, even as it takes a heavy toll.
The signs and symptoms of stress overload can be almost anything. Stress affects the mind, body, and behavior in many ways, and everyone experiences stress differently[1]

Signs and symptoms of stress overload

The following table lists some of the common warning signs and symptoms of stress. The more signs and symptoms you notice in yourself, the closer you may be to stress overload[1]

Stress Warning Signs and Symptoms

Cognitive Symptoms	Emotional Symptoms
• Memory problems • Inability to concentrate • Poor judgment • Seeing only the negative • Anxious or racing thoughts • Constant worrying	• Moodiness • Irritability or short temper • Agitation, inability to relax • Feeling overwhelmed • Sense of loneliness and isolation • Depression or general unhappiness
Physical Symptoms	Behavioral Symptoms
• Aches and pains • Diarrhea or constipation • Nausea, dizziness • Chest pain, rapid heartbeat • Loss of sex drive • Frequent colds	• Eating more or less • Sleeping too much or too little • Isolating yourself from others • Procrastinating or neglecting responsibilities • Using alcohol, cigarettes, or drugs to relax • Nervous habits (e.g. nail biting, pacing)

How much stress is too much?

Because of the widespread damage stress can cause, it's important to know your own limit. But just how much stress is "too much" differs from person to person. Some people roll with the punches, while others crumble at the slightest obstacle or frustration. Some people even seem to thrive on the excitement and challenge of a high-stress lifestyle.

Your ability to tolerate stress depends on many factors, including the quality of your relationships, your general outlook on life, your emotional intelligence, and genetics[2]

Causes of stress

The situations and pressures that cause stress are known as *stressors*. We usually think of stressors as being negative, such as an exhausting work schedule or a rocky relationship. However, anything that puts high demands on you or forces you to adjust can be stressful. This includes positive events such as getting married, buying a house, going to college, or receiving a promotion.

What causes stress depends, at least in part, on your perception of it. Something that's stressful to you may not faze someone else; they may even enjoy it. For example, your morning commute may make you anxious and tense because you worry that traffic will make you late. Others, however, may find the trip relaxing because they allow more than enough time and enjoy listening to music while they drive[3]

Common external causes of stress

- Major life changes
- Work
- Relationship difficulties
- Financial problems
- Being too busy
- Children and family

Common internal causes of stress

Not all stress is caused by external factors. Stress can also be self-generated:

- Inability to accept uncertainty
- Pessimism
- Negative self-talk
- Unrealistic expectations
- Perfectionism
- Lack of assertiveness

Effects of chronic stress

The body doesn't distinguish between physical and psychological threats. When you're stressed over a busy schedule, an argument with a friend, a traffic jam, or a mountain of bills, your body reacts just as strongly as if you were facing a life-or-death situation. If you have a lot of responsibilities and worries, your emergency stress response may be "on" most of the time. The more your body's stress system is activated, the harder it is to shut off.

Long-term exposure to stress can lead to serious health problems. Chronic stress disrupts nearly every system in your body. It can raise blood pressure, suppress the immune system, increase the risk of heart attack and stroke, contribute to infertility, and speed up the aging process. Long-term stress can even rewire the brain, leaving you more vulnerable to anxiety and depression[4]

Many health problems are caused or exacerbated by stress, including:

- Pain of any kind
- Heart disease
- Digestive problems
- Sleep problems
- Depression
- Obesity
- Autoimmune diseases
- Skin conditions, such as eczema

The Need for Stress Management:

Women

Women, in these days, have a lot of balancing to do between home and workplace, including balancing between social and personal requirements. The issues of maternity, menopause, parenthood, gender roles, conditions at home and workplace, familial and social support et al, often blight women`s lives in the long run[5]

Social and Work Stress

Sociological researches assert that family structure (working or stay-at-home mothers and other models) affects performance and employee attendance either directly or interactively. Family demands and family attitudes were found to influence the absence frequency at workplaces.

Experiencing a high level of burnout was associated with increased absenteeism if employees had children under six living at home or reported having difficulty with their child care arrangements. There is a strong relationship between social support and mental stress and trauma in women. It relates to a woman`s help-seeking attitude, social networks, kinship networks, and support networks. Besides these factors, adapting to a new workplace culture and reformations tends in job sectors, affects men and women alike[6]

Gender Role Quantity and quality of leisure time distribution between the genders is an interesting index of how women get burdened with stress for either natural or social obligations. Multinational Time Budget Data Archive and the Australian Time Use Survey suggest that women are now bearing a "dual burden" as both family providers and family carers. Although men and women have similar quantities of free time, when the character of leisure is considered the gap between genders reemerges. Absence of reciprocal and joint emotion management within family is a nagging stressor for women. Mostly mothers handle the bulk of the parental responsibility such as educational and emotional care of children. This can be physically both and psychologically draining.

Stress management has become a big deal today. It is like a demon at our door-step. We never heard of it so much a few years back. But now everyone is talking about it. Today stress has become a condition of living -- a condition that cannot be eliminated from life. It's high time each one of us learn to manage it. Stress is not always bad. In fact, a minimum level of stress is required to lead a productive and a creative life. But if it surpasses the required and manageable level, the consequences can be highly counter-productive and even fatal. Capacity for stress tolerance varies from individual to individual. No absolute standard exists for that[7]

Stress identification and management has a special relevance for doctors who face multiple environmental challenges and demands, tremendous professional accountability, intense Work pressure and patient overload, medical ethics; legal issues on one hand and concern for people and morality on the other, exposing them consistently to stress-prone situations. Combined with these is the challenge that they have to deal with managing the family and their own personal lives. It has been recognized long back that stress could prove very dangerous fordoctors. Doctors are reported to have higher level of stress than among the general population. Doctors have significant psychological vulnerabilities and are more likely to suffer from one or more of the three Ds- drugs, drinks and depression and even suicide than average persons. Doctors who are in general practice seem to be even worse victims of stress. It has been found that about half suffer moderate to severe stress. What makes the situation worse?

Is their reluctance to seek help from professionals in case of any psychological problem? Reluctance to seek help is a major problem.

In Australia, those doctors who neglect the early symptoms of stress and indulge in self-medication have to present themselves before the

Medical Practitioners Board. Stress among general practitioners in Britain also is a regular feature. In addition to personal distress, stress among GPs in England is a great concern because of the problems with recruitment and retention of people required to complete the National Health Scheme led primary healthcare targets. A recent survey on GPs' retirement revealed that a quarter of professionals decided to retire before reaching 60 due to 'health, including stress' which contributed to 36% of these decisions. In 2001, another study showed that 33% of doctors retired due to psychiatric illness[8]

Aims and Objectives

➤ Primary objective is to find the causes of stress in lady doctors of public and private sector hospitals in district Peshawar
➤ To compare the stress between different age groups
➤ To find out the relation of marriage to job and the resultant stress
➤ To assess the environmental factors which influence the occupation directly or indirectly
➤ To Suggest and recommend preventive measures against the risk factors predisposing to stressful environment

HYPOTHESIS

HO: Stress is not caused by different factors in lady doctors of public and private sector hospitals of district Peshawar which are given below:

- Workload,
- Non-cooperation of the patients
- Tiresome job
- Peer pressure from colleagues
- Social obligations
- Hostile environment
- Self-criticism

- Triad of exhaustion, depersonalization and low productivity
- Burden of administration
- Non supporting staff
- Low income
- Lack of time and recognition
- Risk factors of diseases
- Fed up of studies and exams
- Feeling of insecurity
- Non cooperative husband
- Burden of children
- Satisfaction of household chores

H1: Stress is caused by the factors mentioned in H0.

LITERATURE REVIEW

Systematic review of papers reporting suicides in European or North American doctors describes the relative risks of suicides among doctors compared with general population as lying between 1.1 to 3.4 times for male doctors. Reports from the British Medical Association and other researches reveal that 23% of GPs have increased their drinking in response to stress. The consequences of stress on practice has been reported as: prescribing, increased staff turnover, limited team working, increased number of patients' complaints, poor time-keeping and sickness absence, resistance to change or adoption of new technology or systems, disruption in the practice organization, practice partnership split, disloyalty, less motivated or effective staff, little energy and capacity for listening and empathy with patients, problems in relationship with the family, weak communication with patients, withdrawal and isolation. The rate for female doctors is even higher at 2.27 times in relation to the general public. British researchers have also reported doctor's tendency to compulsivity and perfectionism. This is coupled with a type of personality that is highly self-critical. One important manifestation of this perfectionism is the need to portray a healthy image to both patients as well as colleagues due to the perception that good health and doctors are linked with professional medical competence. This is both stressful and a barrier to appropriate self-care. It has been found that the worries about confidentiality and image lead to high levels of self-prescriptions and medication among GPs' high levels of working when sick, and, a low use of formal medical services. The British Medical Association (health policy and economic research unit) passed a resolution in 1998 asking for a report to be prepared on stress among doctors. The aim of the report was to review the research on work-related stress among consultants and GPs. Peer reviews and published studies were located using Medline and by following up relevant citations from retrieved papers. 'Grey literature' such as research reports by relevant organizations was also sought. The British Medical Association has in the past addressed the subjects of stress in the medical profession and the morbidity and mortality of doctors (1993)[9]

This report indicated that there is a large body of evidence that many senior female doctors suffer high levels of stress as result of their work and that this impairs their health and compromises their ability to provide high quality care to their patients. The main source of work-related stress for consultants and GPs is the workload, especially the effect this has on personal life. Other sources of stress are organizational changes, poor management and insufficient resources to do the job, dealing with the patient, sufferings, mistakes, complaints and litigations. Observations point out that stress has become endemic in general practice too. Screening Australian doctors for anxiety and depression using the super general health questionnaires has revealed a high level of stress among female GPs. Similarly, in New Zealand severe stress symptoms are much higher among female GPs than amongst the general population. The troubled doctors group is at risk of becoming 'impaired' in due course[9]

Studies in England have revealed that wives of GPs are four times more likely to commit suicide than other women. Also, it has been observed that main stressors for GPs' spouses are the GPs Detachment from family, communication problems and concern about workload. Stress and suicide among doctors have been even more a matter of grave concern at the global level. Suicide mortality in doctors is reported to be significantly higher in relation to other professionals and general population in many industrialized countries including the US. American doctors kill themselves at a rate of 41% higher comparatively to other places[10]

 The case in India is no better. Four incidents of suicides by female doctors in the recent past have sent out the signals of alarm among the fraternity and common public. In January, 2003-2004 one doctor from the National Institute of Health and Family Welfare (NIHFW) doing diploma in public health committed suicide by hanging herself. On January 24, 2002, one doctor at the Safdar Jung Hospital allegedly committed suicide. He was doing a diploma in Anesthesia, and was a second year student. He injected some poisonous substance to kill himself. Another doctor doing some super general specialty course from the AIIMS committed suicide on July 13, 2004. In February 2005, a senior resident doctor attempted suicide inside his room at the AIIMS. Though these cases have been alarming definitely not surprising. Newspapers frequently report such incidents[11]

Cooper et. al (1989) in their study found four most important predictors of job stress of female GPs work-home interface, demands of the job and patients expectations and practice administration. For women doctors, the most important predictor is the interference of job with the family and for men it is the joint stressors of practice administration and job demands. Most stress come from night calls, emergencies during surgeries and interruption of family life. Stressors for females are identified too. Female doctors experience more stress than their male counterparts from visiting during adverse weather conditions, and fear of being assault on night visits among others. Finding a locum, the working conflict between their work and personal lives, self-medication and less likely to seek formal medical help. Cooper and others have also identified the stressors like high expectations of others, adverse publicity by the media, the working environment, dealing with problem patients, worrying about complaints and arranging hospital admissions and dealing with terminal illness[8]

A study was conducted in Britain by Appleton et. al (1998) on GPs' psychological distress. General health questionnaire-12 (GHQ-12) was used. GHQ-12 was used as a self-report questionnaireto measure psychological symptoms in GPs. Results reported that 52% of respondents scored above the cut-off usually used to diagnose the vulnerable cases of psychiatric morbidity in general population surveys. The results indicated roughly two times more problems among GPs in comparison the general population[1]

Earlier, a similar study was taken up in England by Edwards et. al in 2002. General health questionnaire 28 was administered. Approximately 50% of GPs scored 'as being stressed' which was also twice comparison to the general public. The scores of GPs, however, were comparable with hospital consultants and hospital managers[12]

Howie et. al (1992) carried out studies on occupational stress in GPs, especially in connection with respective timing of consultations and doctors working styles. Many of the main stressors for GPs seemed to be created by their own policies over booking patients, starting surgeries late, accepting commitment too soon after surgeries are due to finish, making insufficient allowances for extra emergency patients and allowing inappropriate telephone calls or other interruptions. Howie and others (1992) in another survey reported that a changing trend in England was the rise of 'inappropriate patient demands' along with 'increasing expectations of what doctors can provide' as a cause of stress, rather than simply an increase in the numbers of patient demands[3]

Pullen et. al (1995) conducted a postal survey of 2,564 doctors. The results revealed that 19% had marital disturbance, 18% emotional disorders, 3% alcohol problems and 1% drug abuse. As many as 26% doctors suffered from one or other medical condition war ranting medical consultation but felt inhibited about consulting a doctor; up to 25% would treat them or not seek treatment for such conditions as alcohol and drug abuse or excessive tiredness and 45% for insomnia and sexual difficulty. Also 76% had self-prescribed antibiotics, 45% non-narcotic analgesics, 35% NSAIDs and 2% had narcotics[13]

Cozens (1997) conducted a study named 'New research on stress in doctors' to find out individual and organizational predictors of stress, depression, alcoholism and early retirement to relate this to performance/error and also to look into individual and organizational interventions. It was a longitudinal study including 318, 4th year students from 1983. They were followed up in 1985, 1993 and 1999. The purpose was to explore long-term predictors of stress, depression, alcoholism and specialty. The study also involved longitudinal study of 126 pre-registration house officers with different types of rotations; study of all general practitioners over 45 in Northeast England, exploring predictors of early retirement; study of all senior registrars in Northeast England exploring training, stress and gender/specialty differences. Stress and depression levels were measured by GHQ and SCL respectively[14]

It was a series of studies with three-fold objectives: 1) to identify individual and organizational predictors of stress, depression, alcoholism and early retirement; 2) to find out its relation to performance/error, to explore individual and organizational interventions. Results of the study indicated that i) stress, depression and indulgence in alcohol are high in doctors; ii) they retire early due to stress and dissatisfaction; iii) all these factors act as hurdles in effective patient care in terms of tiredness, pressured by overwork and depression or anxiety; iv) effects of alcohol; v) decision-making and concentration gets affected by more than half the working day performance during depression; vi) stress and depression lead to more performance related errors; vii) highly stressed are more self-critical; viii) consistency is high, from the first postgraduate year; ix) individual causes include gender, family, career choice, coping and personality; x) gender: women are more depressed than men mainly after graduation, but they are less stressed than men. Female doctors have an increased risk of suicide compared to general population; xi) family in the proportions scoring higher than the threshold on the GHQ for males/females with and without children, fathers and mothers scored higher than others; xii) career choice: surgeons have low stress, depression and high job satisfaction. Psychiatrists and laboratory personnel have high depression. Psychiatrists also have high stress and job dissatisfaction. All these affective states were present as students also; and xiii) among the work/organizational factors of senior doctors dealing with complaints against self, fear of making mistakes and litigation, threat of violence, overwork, conflicts between career and personal life and poor team membership

Interventions have been suggested at individual and organizational level towards creating cost- effective approach to better patient care through healthier staff[14]

Manus et. al (1997-2000) conducted a study on 'Emotional exhaustion and stress in doctors' with the objective of diagnosing the relationship between stress and burnout. A stratified sample of 800 doctors was selected at random from the British medical directory, which has the list of all registered doctors in Britain. Their stress levels were monitored for three years. The sample constituted men and women; and hospital doctors and family practitioners who had qualified between 1950-59 and 1990-94. One among five doctors in each age, sex and practice had qualified outside Britain. The stress level was measured by a 12 item version of GHQ and burn out with Maslach Burn out Inventory including sub-scales on emotional exhaustion, de-personalization (cynicism) and personal accomplishment (professional efficiency). As many as 551 doctors who filled the questionnaire in 1997 were asked to do again three years later in 2000; and 382 (69%) responded. The study findings reveal a reciprocal causation between emotional exhaustion and stress. The largest causal effects in the model showed a causal cycle in which high levels of stress caused emotional exhaustion (b=0.175). Increased levels of personal accomplishment increased stress levels (b=0.080) whereas depersonalization- perceiving patients more as objects than humans lowered stress levels (b=0.105)[2]

Schattner et. al (1998) conducted a study on the 'Stress of metropolitan general practice' by a postal survey of the metropolitan doctors from all states in Victoria. As many as 464 GPs were surveyed with a 64%

response rate (296 participants). Results showed that 13% of GPs had scores suggestive of severe psychiatric disturbance and 30% had mild psychiatric symptoms. Major stressors in descending order were workload, economic factors, medico-political factors, clinical factors, effects of work on outside life, physical working environment. As many as 53% considered leaving general practice because of work stress[15]

Burbeck et. al (2002) conducted a study on 'Occupational stress in consultants in accident and emergency medicine: a national survey of levels of stress at work. The objective was to assess levels of occupational stress amongst the British accident and emergency consultants. The method used was postal survey. The results indicated that 154 respondents had GHQ-12 scores over the threshold for distress. Levels of depression as measured by the SCL-D were 18%, slightly higher than other groups. About 34 (10%) reported suicidal ideation. Women had significantly higher SCL-D scores than men. Respondents were highly satisfied with A&E as a specialty. Protective factors found in other occupational groups did not apply. Only one demographic or work-related factor, number of time posts significantly correlated with either stress outcome measure. Logistic regression modeling revealed 'being overstretched', 'effect of hours and stress on family life', and 'lack of recognition' were significant predictors of GHQ identified cases, while 'the effect of stress on family life', low prestige of specialty, and 'dealing with management' predicted SCL-D scores[4]

 A British Medical Audit Advisory Group conducted a survey in 1993 on the 'Causes of Stress in GPs'. The causes identified were rank ordered as emergency calls during surgery hours, night calls, time pressure, working after a sleepless night, dealing with problem patients, worrying about patient complaints, interruption of family life, 24-hour responsibility for patients' lives and unrealistically high expectations by others of the doctors role and partner on a holiday[16]

Vanagas and Alxelsson (2004) conducted a cross-sectional study on 'Interaction among GPs age and patient load, prediction of job strain, decision latitude and perception demands – across sectional study'. It was a study done through a mailed survey of random national sample. Computerized sampling was performed from the registry of the Lithuanian physicians. Total number of GPs in Lithuania at that time was 1,007. Out of this, 300 Lithuanian GPs were chosen[17]

Psychosocial stress was investigated with the questionnaire based on the Reeder scale. Job demands were investigated on the Karasek scale. The analysis included descriptive statistics: logistic regression Beta coefficients to find out the predictors and interactions between characteristics and predictors. Work characteristics were measured by the Karasek ' Job Content Questionnaire. This has two scales that measure stressful job character – job decision latitude and psychosocial workload demands. This model is also known as the 'job strain' model. Psychological workload demands were defined by questions such as 'working very fast, very hard', 'doing so many things'. Job decisions latitude was measured with questions as: 'always must learn for new and working a lot'. A four-point Liker-like scale was used with the coding from 4-1 for series. Results revealed that Lithuanian GPs have high patient load and are at risk of stress, they have high job demands and decision latitude. Jobs train development and higher job demands can be influenced in duration of general practice. However, older GPs perceived less strain[17]

Sharma (2005) conducted a study on 'Role stress among doctors'. Role stress was measured by Pareek's Psychological Instrument. Ten (10) role stresses included in the study were: i) inter-role distance (IRD): focuses on conflicts between organizational and non-organizational roles; ii) role stagnation (RS): focuses on feeling of getting stuck in one role; iii) role expectation conflict (REC): focuses on conflicting expectations of various important people in the office like supervisors, subordinates and peer group; iv) role erosion (RE): focuses on the feeling that role occupant's functions are being performed by someone else; v) role overload (RO): focuses on the feeling that expectations from the role occupant are many; vi) role isolation (RI): focuses on the psychological distance between one's role and role of others in the same role set; vii) personal inadequacy (PI): focuses on the feelings of incompetence on part of the role occupant; viii) self-role distance (SRD): focuses on the feeling that demands of one's role are in conflict with one's self- concept; ix) role ambiguity (RA): focuses on lack of clarity about role expectation; and x) resource inadequacy (RIn): focuses on the feelings of the role occupant that he has not been given adequate resources[18]

Spurgeon et. al (2005) in a study on stress among GPs found that older practitioners were more stressed by the new contract demands in comparison to younger doctors, but younger doctors were more stressed by unrealistic patient demands. Those GPs who considered the job stress responsible for causing them psychological symptoms of ill health were those who reported being particularly stressed about the effects of work on their homes and social lives. Worrying about patients' complaints was an important stressor as was a feeling that the media was becoming more hostile and creating a blame culture[19]

Irene Van Ham et. al (2006) conducted their study from 1990 to 2006. In their results, they found 24 relevant citations. Factors increasing job satisfaction which were mentioned more than twice were: diversity of work, relations and contact with colleagues, and being involved in teaching medical students. Factors decreasing job satisfaction were: low income, too many working hours, administrative burdens, heavy workload, lack of time, and lack of recognition[20]

Dambisya (2004) has reported that "little information exists on the career paths and destinations of graduates of medical schools from developing countries, in contrast with many such reports from the developed world". Women have been historically found lacking in administrative role and hospital administration appears historically as a male profession predominantly (Borkowski and Walsh, 1992). Green et al. (2004) have argued that gender is still a major issue in the workplace because of the impact that gender stereotypes have on the attitudes and decision making of employers and employees alike. Moreover, satisfaction with career is also aligned with practicing male norms (Broadbridge, 2007) because obstacles often impede women's career paths more than men's (Madsen and Blide, 1992). Moreover, perceptions by women and men of a woman as homemaker and mother create serious conflicts when jobs are demanding and time intensive Madsen and Blide (1992) and if they wish to advance, they may have to move to nontraditional work settings (Robinson, 2004; Baruch,2006; Swanson and Fouad, 2009). Education is also expected to influence one's beliefsconcerning one's marketability. Human capital theory states, "More educated workers havemore options because they have increased their human capital investment" (Wayne et al., 1999: 580). Hence, the doctors today demand significantly different lifestyle desiring to keep leisure and work separate and balanced (Ek et al., 2005) requiring better personal and time management skills. Doctors, in fact are seeking careers that involve less occupational stress while having a potential for 'controllable lifestyle' (Ek et al., 2005)[21]

Mangan (2009) has described lady doctors' career as "leaking pipeline" because of their shying away from 'academic medicine' and other highly demanding professional careers. Research has evidenced that women are more likely to be found in less prestigious and lower income specialties such as pediatrics, obstetrics gynecology, psychiatry, pathology and family practice (Jagsi et al., 2007) and they are prepared for under-representation in top positions in medical organizations and medical school facilities. Though many female physicians marry either other physicians or highly career oriented Professionals, still they fail to follow a smooth career path. If women are to move through the glass ceiling, health care institutions must become sensitized to the factors that prevent women's advancement and facilitate entry-level opportunities for women in administration (Davidson and Cooper, 1992; Hamel et al., 2006)[22]

Yasmeen (2005) has identified that due to cultural and traditional practices even highly educated women did not receive equal rights as those of men in traditional society of Pakistan. She (Yasmeen) has advocated for an awareness campaign about harmful traditional practices based on the idea of the inferiority or superiority of either sex or on stereotyped roles ofgender at all levels in society to modify the social and cultural attitudes of both men and women in Pakistan[23]

Bickel and Clark (2000) have noted that women receive inadequate mentoring and encouragement in their career development or partly because of women's tendency to think of relationships in terms of support and affiliation, whereas men are more accustomed to competition and hierarchy, which is the tendency to view relationships in professional, educational and/or workplace context. Nizami et al., (2006) have discussed that multiple factors can influence a person's level of job satisfaction; these factors range from the level of pay and benefits, perceived fairness of the promotion system within the organization, the quality of theworking conditions to leadership and social relationships. Furthermore, they (Nizami et al.) have pointed out lack of communication and cooperation between professionals as major sources of distress and dissatisfaction among female doctors. Bano et al. (2005) has identified the source of stress for lady doctors in Pakistan, which tends to multiply, occupational stress into family stress[24]

OB Familoni et. al (2005) in their study found many different causes of stress among female GPs. Some of them are listed: Specific stressors include Peer pressure- within the profession and across professions.Social expectation- The doctor is still perceived as a very comfortable person in our society and expectations are usually high financially and otherwise. Failure or inability to 'meet up' may constitute a significant stress factor in some physicians.Training-at both the undergraduate and postgraduate levels are long and tedious. Getting into the few medical schools is like passing through the proverbial eye of the needle, yet the remunerations and the social acceptability and recognition are not commensurate.Hostile Job Environment- Administrative ineptitude and bureaucratic bottlenecks can make the job situation very frustrating. Inadequate infrastructure, unavailable and obsolete equipments make the long years and fortune spent in training at home and abroad a waste. Unsecured future, delays in promotion and inappropriate capacity utilization are some of the causes of unfulfilment and stress in the job place. Long working hours was specifically identified in the BMA report. This could be compounded in our environment by denied and 'monetized' holidays, sometimes because of manpower shortages and/or poverty. Inadequate personal training and retraining, and lack of continuous education can lead to loss of self-esteem and frustration in our profession where changes and development go on at jet speed. Fear of mistakes and litigations are becoming increasingly important.The 'burnt out phenomenon', a terminology made popular by Felton (11) consists of a triad of emotional exhaustion, depersonalization (treating patients and other people as if they were objects) and low productivity/achievements. It is particularly common in health professionals under stress. These invariably lead to 'impairment of health, grief and suffering'. It compromises the quality of care which may lead to litigation and a vicious cycle. In some cases it may lead to premature retirement due to physical and/or mental health. Premature death, even by suicide is a distinct possibility[7]

Brewin et. al (1997) conducted a 2 year study on both male and female doctors. They found that self-criticism was the significant predictor of stress among lady doctors[25]

N. Krishna Reddyet. al (2010) studied the nature of specific strains and stresses among married women in their marital, occupational and house work roles. They found that strains and stresses are lower in family roles than in occupational and household roles among the married women. These have more severe consequences for the psychological well-being of women than occupational strains and stresses. Strains predicted distress through role-specific stress, with strains deriving from contribution of role-specific stress[26]

Jenny Firth Cozens et. al (1998) in their study found out that relationships with senior doctors andpatients are the main reported stressors, followed by making mistakes and conflict of career with personal life. The predictors of symptom levels varied for men and women. In men, depression and self-criticism as students, and current sleep levels; and in women, sibling rivalry and current alcohol use, were the main predictors: in men, 27% of the variance was accounted for by early dispositional factors alone compared with 14% in women. A model is suggested linking sleep loss with workplace stressors, self-critical cognitions, and depression[25]

Syed Shakir Ali Ghazali et. al (2007) in their study found out that overall, 56% doctors were not satisfied and only 10% are very much satisfied with the level of their income. Among those very much satisfied, 60% are those having M.Phil. or FCPS degree. Among those having MBBS/ BDS degree, 65% are not satisfied with the level of their income. Among M.Os/ Registrars/ Demonstrators, 70.59% are not satisfied with the level of their income, whereas only 20% of those working as Assistant Professors above are not satisfied with the level of income. It is found that, 48% of the doctors are not satisfied with their working environment and out of these 83.33% are M.Os. / Registrars/ Demonstrators. Only 6% are really satisfied with their working environment. Among those working as Assistant Professors or above, 20% are not satisfied with the working environment. 92% of all the doctorsare not satisfied with the present service structure.All thosehaving MCPS/Diploma are not satisfied whereas 85% of the MBBS/BDS and 94.44% of M.Phil./FCPS are not satisfied with present service structure. 92% of the doctors are not satisfied with the career prospects in Pakistan and out of these 69.57% are M.Os./Registrars/ Demonstrators. None of the Senior Registrar/Assistant Professors are satisfied with their carrier prospectus in Pakistan. The results indicate that 78% of the doctors would like to serve abroad and out of these 74.36% are M.Os / Registrars / Demonstrators. Among those working as Assistant Professors or above, 60% are willing to serve abroad[27]

Fiona Godlee et. al (1990) in her study on female GPs stated that it is children that block career achievement. Full time working women have on average 17 hours a week less leisure time than men, and a recent study of British social attitudes showed that when both parents work full time the woman still takes on most of the child rearing and household tasks: 82% of men and women said that the woman was ultimately responsible for these[28]

Imtiaz et. al (2012) in their study found major problems faced by females particularly among doctors in our society. The problems seem to rise with the chauvinistic, conservative society of Pakistan; hence itdoes not offer equal educational opportunities to women in all fields. Many women desirous of pursuing higher education are forced to choose either medicine or education as their specialty despite their aptitude and interest in other fields. The obvious outcome is that they are not keen to practice medicine afterwards. In many families the prevalent trend is to become a doctor solely to get the title and status. Parents believe that their daughters would get better suitors if they are doctors. Women are not expected to be the head of a family or the bread earner therefore the drive to work progress and attain a better socio economic status is missing in female physicians. Female physicians lack role models in our society and they are not as goal oriented as their counterparts are. They are in constant battle with the odds and often end up contributing much less than their true potential. After a woman gets married, lots of responsibilities welcome her. Her life changes altogether. In these circumstances it becomes extremely difficult for her to continue with her profession. Most female physician drop outs complain that they had to abandon their jobs because their spouse and in-laws pressurized them to do so. The uncooperative attitude of the family and their constant demand from a woman to be a home maker and professional simultaneously puts her in a great dilemma. Notwithstanding the stress, most women sacrifice their professional life and opt to become the "lady of the house". When a female's role changes to that of a mother's, her priorities change. Considering family obligations to be the first priority, a woman has to sacrifice her other skills. Some may sail through these difficult times with the help of an extended family but in the troubled times of the modern era the concept of joint family system is fast fading. In a research conducted on problems of female doctors working in hospital in Pakistan District Faisalabad, 70% responded with having problems looking after children with job. A woman starts losing her ongoing battle of maintaining a balance between motherhood and her profession because her employers don't provide adequate facilities catering to her needs e.g. both public and private sector hospitals sanction only a maternity leave of 12 weeks which is quite less when compared with that offered to women in developed countries. Similarly there are hardly any day care centers in hospitals in Pakistan. The increased workload is a major cause of dissatisfaction among female physicians. Another discouraging factor is the harassment faced by lady doctors in the streets and in workplaces. A bill called the "The

Protection against Harassment of Women at the Workplace Act 2010"
was passed but the compliance has been low and women are still facing
skeptic and biased attitudes at the hands of investigators and
disciplinary committees when they make complaints against the
violence they face. The society at large doesn't accept female
physicians in specialties outside the domain of gynecology, obstetrics
and pediatrics. The population fails to show its confidence in female
physicians especially when it comes to handling emergency situations
and surgical procedures. There is gender discrimination and this is
becoming a major hurdle in the path of women desirous of exploring
the different avenues of medicine. Still unkind is the attitude of the
government towards female physicians. No incentives are provided
whatsoever. The meager pay scale and shaggy work places serve only
to dampen the spirit and enthusiasm of young female physicians. The
unavailability of jobs with flexible working hours disrupts the balance
maintained by the "super woman" juggling her personal and
professional life[29]

METHODOLOGY

STUDY DESIGN:

This was a cross sectional study done over a period of 6 months from March 2013 to August 2013 in four tertiary hospitals of Peshawar out of which two are government run and two are private (Khyber Teaching hospital, Hayatabad Medical Complex, Northwest and Rehman Medical Institute).

SAMPLING TECHNIQUE:

Simple random sampling was used to achieve the required sample size.

STUDY POPULATION:

This includes 200 lady doctors of age group 24-60 from four tertiary care hospitals of Peshawar, half survey done in government hospitals while half of it in private hospitals. We were successful in interviewing 100 lady doctors, half in each sector.

INCLUSION CRITERIA:

All lady doctors working in age group 24-60.

EXCLUSION CRITERIA:

Lady doctors practicing in only walk-in-clinics.

QUESTIONNAIRE:

A well-structured dichotomous questionnaire (yes\no) was designed that consist of questions about sociodemographic information and different stress related questions.

It included:

- Questions were asked about workload, working hours and administration malpractice to evaluate the institution based stress.
- For the evaluation of job related problems, questions were asked about the attitude of the professors, colleagues and other assisting staff.
- Questions were asked about the behavior of husband, children and management of household chores to evaluate family problems.

VARIABLES:

DEPENDENT/OUTCOME VARIABLE:

Stress

INDEPENDENT VARIABLES:

Job Related Problems: Workload, working hours, exhaustion, hostile job environment, lack of time, low salary, risk factors of diseases, exams and studies

Social problems: Social obligations, peer pressure, insecurity

Family problems: Non-cooperative husband, burden of children, management of household chores

DATA MANAGEMENT AND ANALYSIS:

Data was analyzed using SPSS version 20.0. Results were plotted and conclusion drawn.

LIMITATIONS:

The study has been done with a relatively small sample. To make effective generalizations, a longitudinal study with increased sample is suggested. Personal bias may have affected data interpretation and analysis to some extent, though we have tried our best to be self-critical and reflexive to minimize the bias.

RESULTS

Following are the results of factors that influenced the target population each categorized according to the prevalence in specific area (public or private hospital) and its existence in different age groups:

1) **VARIABLES AFFECTINGGOVERNMENT HOSPITALS'
   POPULATION (All age groups i.e. 24-60):**

Work Load

		Frequency	Percent	Valid Percent	Cumulative Percent
Valid	Government	72	72.0	72.0	72.0
	Private	28	28.0	28.0	100.0
	Total	100	100.0	100.0	

Table 1.1

Low Salary

		Frequency	Percent	Valid Percent	Cumulative Percent
Valid	Government	70	70.0	70.0	70.0
	Private	30	30.0	30.0	100.0
	Total	100	100.0	100.0	

Table 1.2

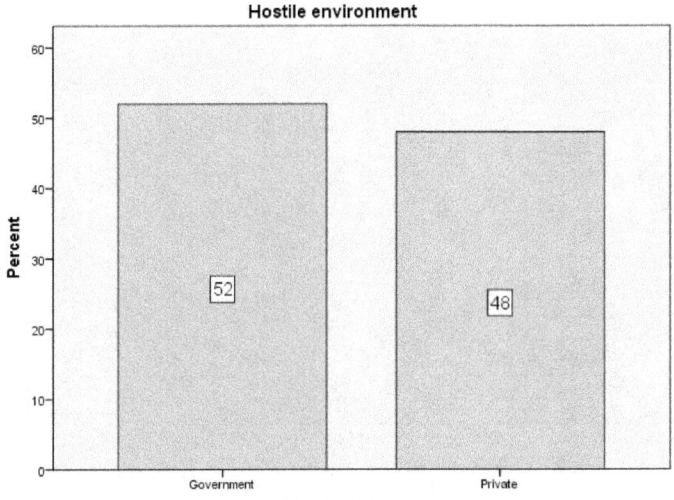

Graph 1.1

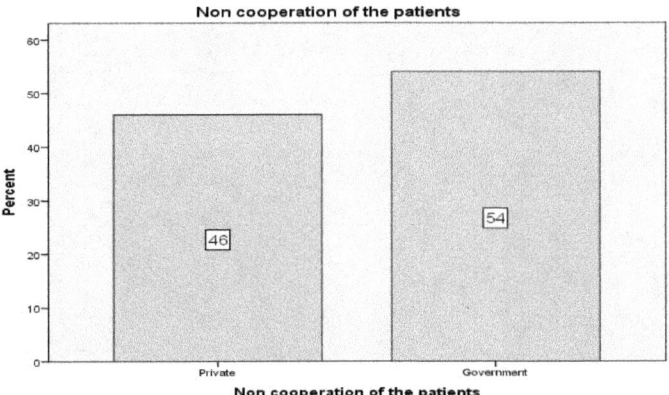

Graph 1.2

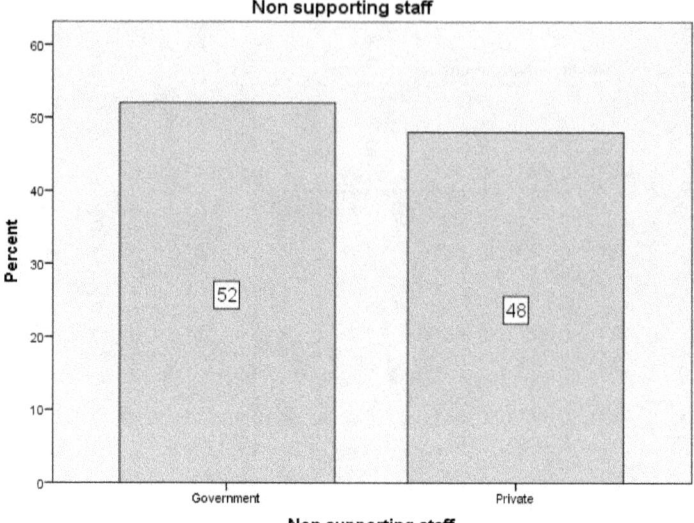

Graph 1.3

2) VARIABLES AFFECTINGPRIVATE HOSPITALS' POPULATION (All age groups i.e. 24-60):

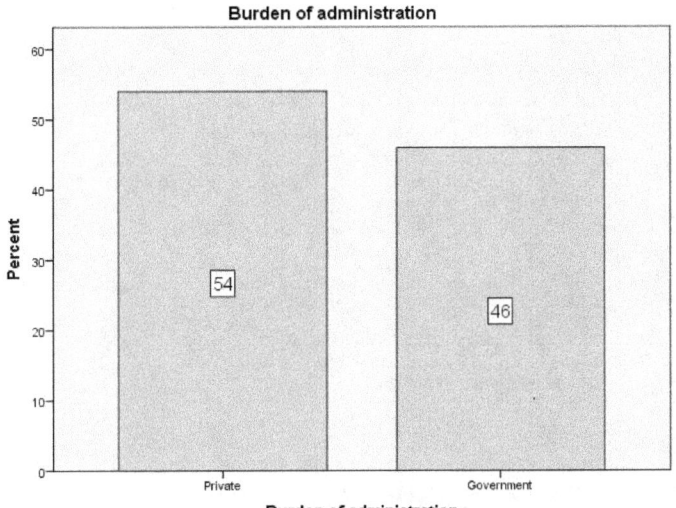

Graph 2.1

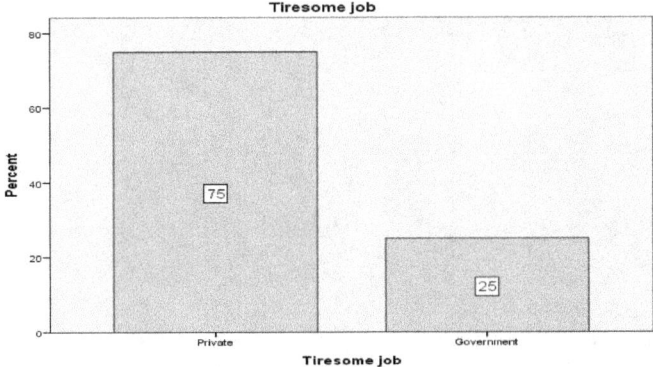

Graph 2.2

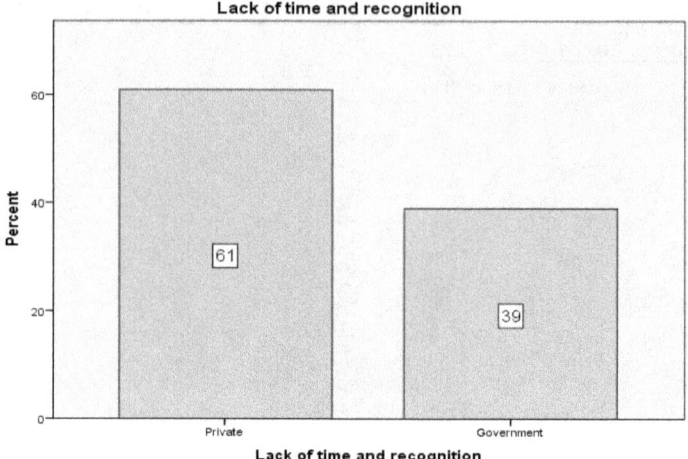

Graph 2.3

3) VARIABLES AFFECTING AGE GROUP 24-30:

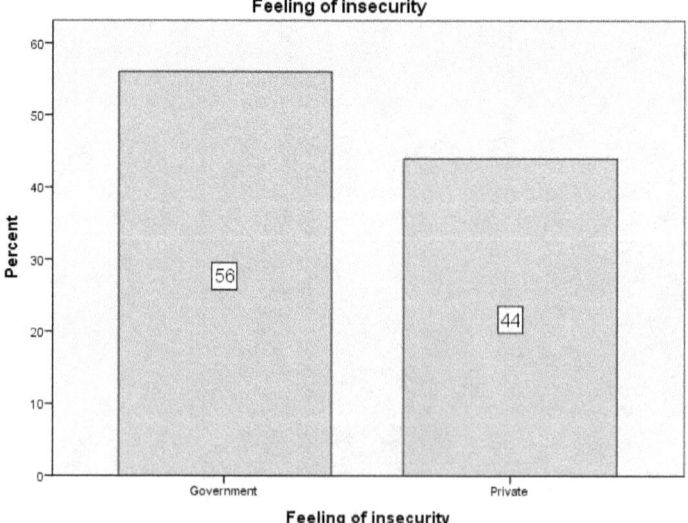

Graph 3.1

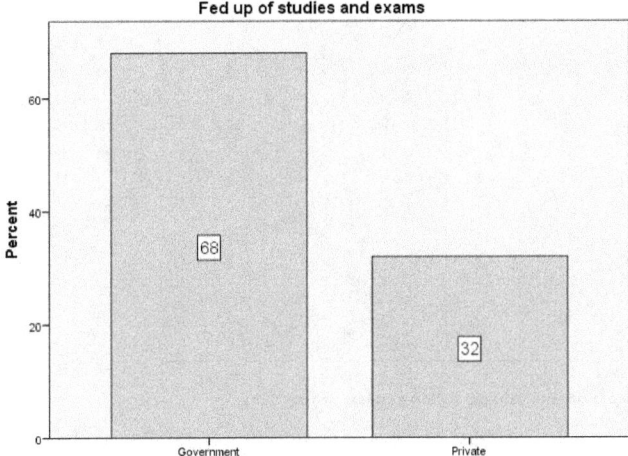

Graph 3.2

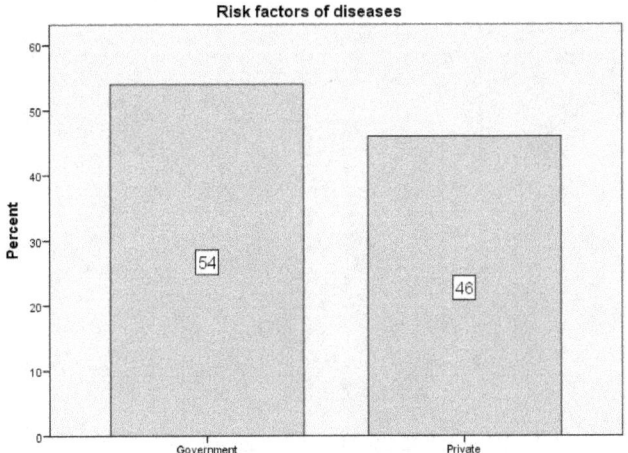

Graph 3.3

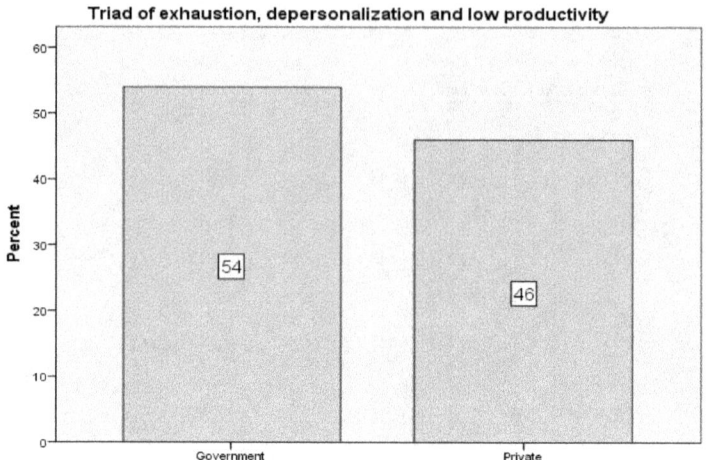

Graph 3.4

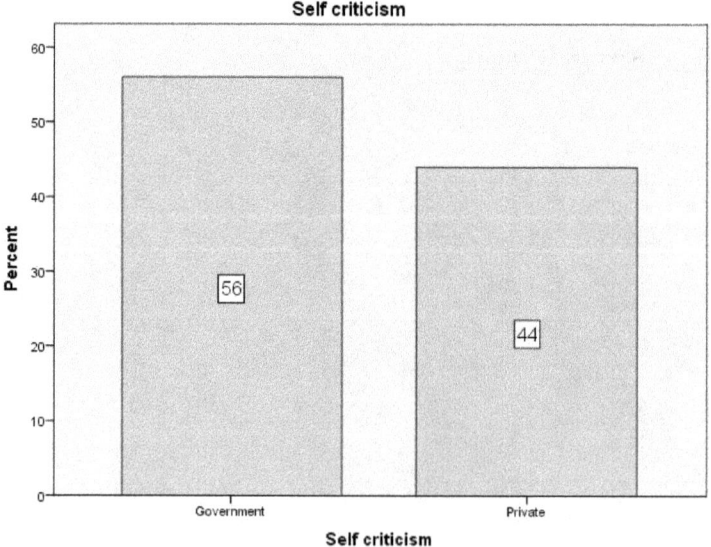

Graph 3.5

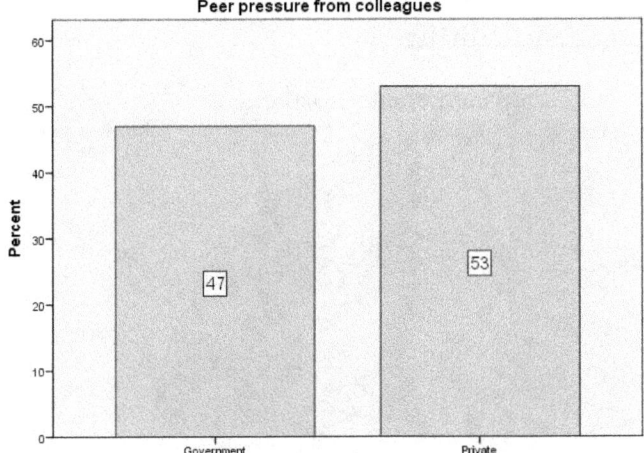

Graph 3.6

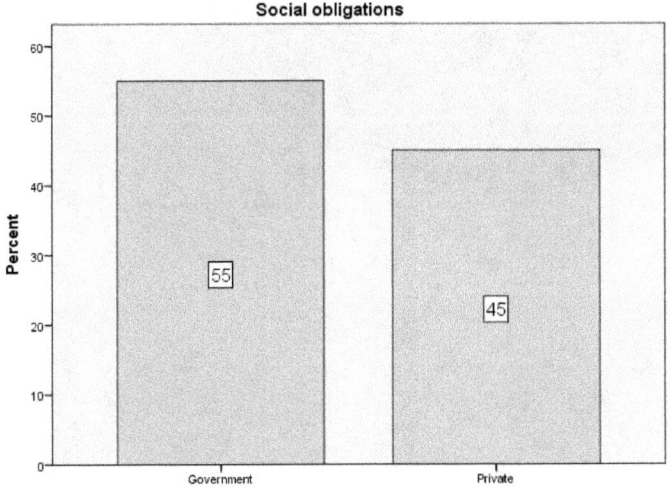

Graph 3.7

4) VARIABLES AFFECTING MARRIED LADY DOCTORS IRRESPECTIVE OF ANY AGE GROUP:

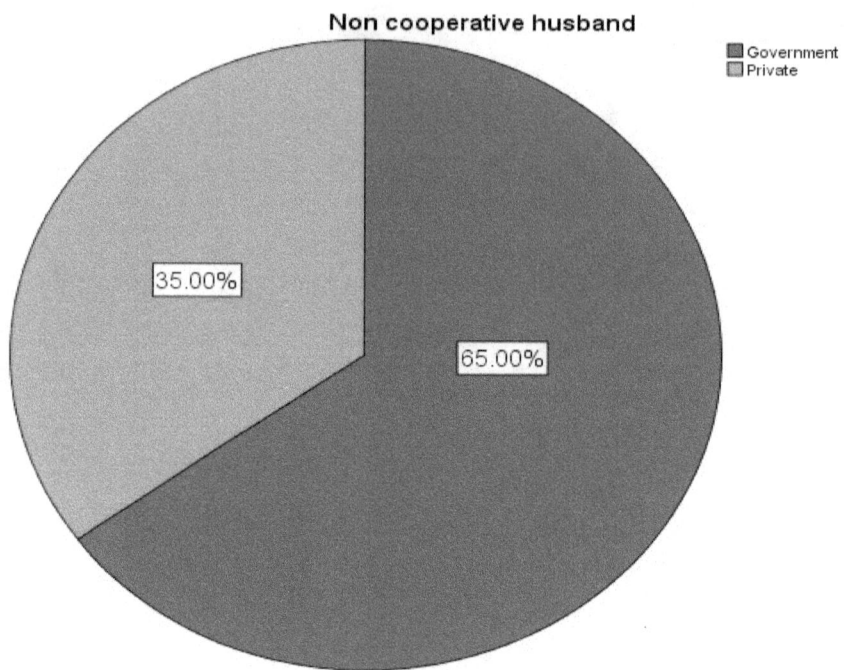

Figure 4.1

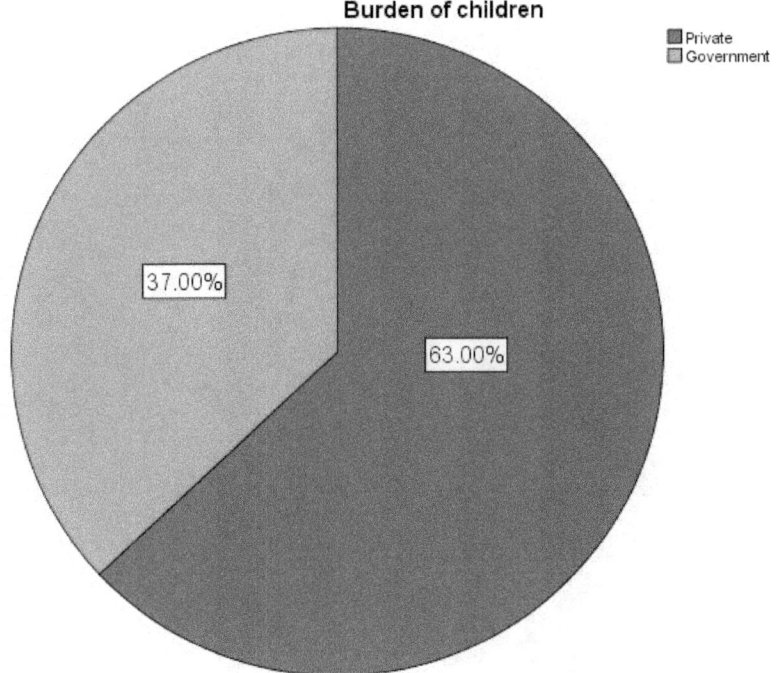

Figure 4.2

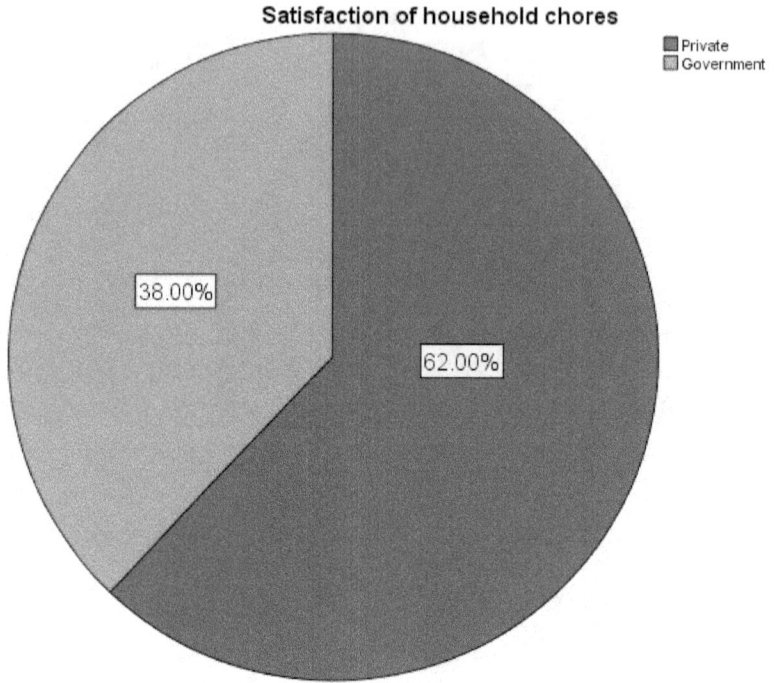

Figure 4.3

DISCUSSION

Workload being the most common stressor was found to be 72% in public sector hospitals while the rate being shockingly low in private hospitals that is about 28%. As a matter of fact, workload was expected to be equally high in both sector hospitals but many lady doctors working in private hospitals seem to have been masked their workload shifts because of handsome amount of salary they get there. Low salary, uncooperative patients, hostile environment and non-supporting staff was found to be 70%, 54%, 52%, and 52% while in private sector it was 30%, 46%, 48 % and 48 %, respectively. Public hospitals usually pay which doesn't suffice the basic standard needs of a working lady doctor. Such hospitals also receive patients that belong to the low socioeconomic part of the society thus its high rate of burden is justified while hostile ambience attributes to the fact that teaching staff doesn't tolerate much of the juvenile mistakes made by residents working under them. Burden of administration, exhaustion and lack of time and recognition were variables found at higher rate in private sect. that are 54%, 75% and 61% respectively. These private sect. exclusive stress factors are based on the fact that private sect. hospitals' agenda is to acquire maximum output from working staff, leaving them with inadequate time for themselves while recruiting fewer doctors, so the burden of administration shifts to the handful amount of staff. Stressors that were found in young doctors from age group 24-30 irrespective of the sector are insecurity, exams and studies stress, vulnerability to diseases, burnt out phenomena, self-criticism, peer pressure and social expectations which rated 56%, 68%, 54%, 54%, 56%, 47% and 55% respectively. Such age group that are newly recruited lady doctors are delicate to the working system, hence they end up in stress. Married workgroup stressors were uncooperative husband, burden of children and satisfaction of household chores which are 65%, 37% and 62% in public hospitals while 35%, 63% and 38% in private hospitals, respectively. Two of these variables' rate is higher in public sect. that is uncooperative husband and dissatisfaction of household chores which maybe be attributed to the fact that lady doctors working in public hospitals are already prone to more stress factors which secondarily affects their marital life as well while those working in private hospitals encounters the problem of raising their children because they are mostly at job and lack of time leads them to worry more and more about their children being abandoned.

CONCLUSION

The occupational life of Pakistani lady doctors is influenced by sociopolitical, cultural and personal variables. Results have suggested that (a) too much workload is being put unevenly on lady doctors of government hospitals; they are given long tiresome shifts with inadequate salaries, the staff being too insolent which directly affects feminine mentality and the patient overload is too much to handle; (b) on the other hand, private sector hospitals put too much administrative responsibilities which leave lady doctors with almost no personal time; (c) the age group 24-30 which accounts for almost the highest strength in any tertiary hospital was effected mostly because of lack of social security, the vulnerability to communicable diseases because of unhygienic working environment and poor maintenance of hospitals, such age groups is also prone to experience stress because of too many social obligations, too many exams to pass and inevitable peer pressure from colleagues; (d) background variables, socioeconomic status, and relocation with family strongly influenced the sense of self and career motivation in married lady doctors. The noncooperation of husbands affected them mostly, while burden of children and household chores exaggerating their stress further.

According to our survey, such stress factors are pretty much manageable. It is a common perception that lady doctors tend to avoid loads of responsibility, search for escapes and show emotional instability in handling critical situations. In order to reach leadership status, they must acquire and polish leadership skills, especially communication and stress management. However, keeping in view the loss of human resource and our cultural constraints, policies need some modification at governmental level to get some relief providing lady doctors protection from unhygienic and un productive occupational stress, offering them equitable salaries, protected time and means of covering small crises at home and at work by flexible hours, freedom to fail, open-minded mentors and collaborators to mend the "leaky pipe" leading to both objective and subjective success in profession and stress free environment.

RECOMMENDATIONS

General:

> - One should give plenty of time to rest and entertainment.
> - Lady doctors should avoid work under too much stress. This could lead to major depression disorder.
> - If possible, should choose to work in institutions where her close friends are working.
> - Always avoid people who stress you out.
> - Share feelings with whom you trust.
> - Learn to forgive and control your anger.
> - Keep your sense of humor active every time.
> - Do something you enjoy every day.
> - Our hospitals and clinics need to be more job-friendly. The various authorities have a responsibility to provide the minimum implements required to perform our duties.
> - The medical curriculum, particularly in developing countries should be strengthened with courses such as administration and financial management.
> - Holidays are refreshing and should be taken at least once a year. The tendency to 'monetize' holidays or pick up a locum job during holiday period should be discouraged.
> - There is need to control excess workload particularly in the junior doctor cadre.

Diet:

- Avoid over eating and under eating.
- Avoid the use of too much caffeine and sugar.
- Eat healthy balance diet which includes more fruits and vegetables.

Government Hospitals:

- Work load should be distributed equally and to the capacity of doctors. A community should be provisioned in order to keep check and balance.
- Wages and salaries should be based on working hours of a doctor. In this way, the person will feel rewarding and doctors will always be motivated to work any hour of the day.
- Head of wards and departments should keep an eye on staff so that female doctors won't face harassment of any kind from any working person at hospital.
- Non cooperative patients should be left at the disposal of head of departments who are quite used to dealing such patients.
- Private hospitals:
- More medical staff should be recruited in order to ease the burden of administration work.
- Working hours should be decreased to the capacity of the doctors.

Young doctors (age group 24-30):

- Strict action should be taken against any kind of immoral and insolent acts of the staff irrespective of the gender. No question of insecurity will rise.

- One should give plenty of time to herself and plan out schedules, so to minimize the work-exams conflict.
- Doctors should wear masks and gloves in order to lessen the risk of acquiring communicable diseases.
- Booster dose vaccination should be done to further immunity against acquiring disease.
- Doctors should give themselves rest whenever they don't have the responsibility of clinical rounds and duties. Exhaustion messes up work.
- One should learn to keep herself contented and avoid self-criticism and overthinking.
- Lady doctors should explore their own limits of carrying out tasks and avoid the habit of getting caught up in the peer pressure of colleagues.
- Young lady doctors should explain their role at home and to her circle so that she is made guilty every time is was unable to fulfill the social obligations and expectations.

Married Lady Doctors:

- Lady doctors should maintain pleasant relationship with her husband even if she is stressed at times. This will help maintain peace between and unnecessary quarrels won't arise. She should make ultimate understand with her hubby so he supports her through every up and down.
- Married doctors can hire a housekeeper to look after her children and carry out the household chores whenever she is away doing her duties at the hospitals in case she could afford one.

REFERENCES

1) Appleton, Kevin, Allan House, and Anthony Dowell. "A survey of job satisfaction, sources of stress and psychological symptoms among general practitioners in Leeds." *The British Journal of General Practice* 48, no. 428 (1998): 1059.

2) Ziv, Stephen D. Small, Paul Root Wolpe, Amitai. "Patient safety and simulation-based medical education." *Medical teacher* 22, no. 5 (2000): 489-495.

3) Matthey, Stephen, David J. Kavanagh, Pauline Howie, Bryanne Barnett, and Margaret Charles. "Prevention of postnatal distress or depression: an evaluation of an intervention at preparation for parenthood classes." *Journal of Affective Disorders* 79, no. 1 (2004): 113-126.

4) Burbeck, R., S. Coomber, S. M. Robinson, and C. Todd. "Occupational stress in

consultants in accident and emergency medicine: a national survey of levels of stress at work." *Emergency Medicine Journal* 19, no. 3 (2002): 234-238.

5) Kumar, Shailesh, Jesse Fischer, Elizabeth Robinson, Simon Hatcher, and R. N. Bhagat. "Burnout and job satisfaction in New Zealand psychiatrists: a national study." *International journal of social psychiatry* 53, no. 4 (2007): 306-316.

6) Feddock, Christopher A., Andrew R. Hoellein, John F. Wilson, Timothy S. Caudill, and Charles H. Griffith. "Do pressure and fatigue influence resident job performance?." *Medical teacher* 29, no. 5 (2007): 495-497.

7) Hall, Martica H. "Behavioral medicine and sleep: Concepts, measures, and methods." In *Handbook of Behavioral Medicine*, pp. 749-765. Springer New York, 2010.

8) Antoniou, Alexandros-Stamatios G., Marilyn J. Davidson, and Cary L. Cooper. "Occupational stress, job satisfaction and health state in male and female junior hospital doctors in Greece." *Journal of Managerial Psychology* 18, no. 6 (2003): 592-621.

9) 1)Wang, JianLi, Scott B. Patten, Shawn Currie, Jitender Sareen, and Norbert Schmitz. "A population-based longitudinal study on work environmental factors and the risk of major depressive disorder." American journal of epidemiology 176, no. 1 (2012): 52-59.

10) 11) Health Policy and Economic Research Unit, author (1998). Work   Related Stress Among Junior Doctors. London: BMA; http://www.pubmedcentral.nih.gov/articlerender.fcgi?artid=2408543

11) Dhar, Neera, U. Datta, and Deoki Nandan. "Stress among doctors–a review." Health and Population: Perspectives and Issues 31,   no.4 (2008): 256_266

12) Calabrese, Edward J., Kenneth A. Bachmann, A. John Bailer, P. Michael Bolger, Jonathan Borak, Lu Cai, Nina Cedergreen et al. "Biological stress response terminology: Integrating the concepts of adaptive response and preconditioning stress within a hormetic dose–response framework." *Toxicology and applied pharmacology* 222, no. 1 (2007): 122-128.

13) Kay, Margaret, Geoffrey Mitchell, Alexandra Clavarino, and Jenny Doust. "Doctors as patients: a systematic review of doctors' health access and the barriers they experience." *The British Journal of General Practice* 58, no. 552 (2008): 501.

14) Firth-Cozens, Jenny. "Individual and organizational predictors of depression in general practitioners."

The British Journal of General Practice 48, no. 435 (1998): 1647

15) Schattner L. Peter and Coman J. Greg (1998) : The Stress of Metropolitan General Practice, MJA; 169: 133-137

16) Clare A. The pain of change. In: Currie E. What women want. ILondon: Sidgwick and Jackson, 1990:255-70

17) Vanagas, Giedrius, and Susanna Bihari-Axelsson. "Interaction among general practitioners age and patient load in the prediction of job strain, decision latitude and perception of job demands. A Cross-sectional study." BMC public Health 4, no. 1 (2004): 59.

18)) Sharma Ekta: Role Stress Among Doctors,(2005) Journal of Health Management, Vol. 7, No. 1, 151- 156.

19)) Spurgeon P, Barwell F and Maxwell R (2005): 'Stress and   General Practice ' : website : www.rcgp.org.uk/pdf/ ISS_ INFO_22_ FEB05.pdf, Royal   College   of Journal Practitioners, February.

20) Van Ham, Irene, Anita AH Verhoeven, Klaas H. Groenier, Johan W. Groothoff, and Jan De Haan. "Job satisfaction among general practitioners: a systematic literature review." European Journal of general practice 12, no. 4 (2006): 174-180.

21) Arif, Seema. "Broken wings: issues faced by female doctors in Pakistan regarding career development." International Journal of Academic Research in Business and Social Sciences 1 (2011): 79-101.

22) Thomason, Timothy. "A Week in the Life of a University Professor: Issues of Stress, Workload, and Wellness." Counseling and Wellness 3 (2012).

23) Ahmed-Little, Yasmin. "Implications of shift work for junior doctors." BMJ: British Medical Journal 334, no. 7597 (2007): 777.

24) Verlander, Glese. "Female physicians: balancing career and family." Academic Psychiatry 28, no. 4 (2004): 331-336.

25) Firth-Cozens, Jenny, and Joanne Greenhalgh. "Doctors' perceptions of the links between stress and lowered clinical care." Social science & medicine 44, no. 7 (1997): 1017-1022.

26) Varadhan, Krishna K., Keith R. Neal, Cornelius HC Dejong, Kenneth CH Fearon, Olle Ljungqvist, and Dileep N. Lobo. "The enhanced recovery after surgery (ERAS) pathway for patients undergoing major elective open colorectal surgery: a meta-analysis of randomized controlled trials." Clinical nutrition 29, no. 4 (2010): 434-440.

27) Shaheen, Kounser, and Riyaz Ahmad Guide Rainayee. "Relation Of Employee Job Satisfaction

And Patient Satisfaction In Select Private Medical Care Centers In Kashmir Valley." PhD diss., 2012.

28) Godlee, Fiona. "Making reviewers visible." JAMA: the journal of the American Medical Association 287, no. 21 (2002): 2762-2765.

29) Mumford, David B., Muhammad Ayub, Raheel Karim, Nasir Izhar, Aftab Asif, and John T. Bavington. "Development and validation of a questionnaire for anxiety and depression in Pakistan." Journal of affective disorders 88, no. 2 (2005): 175-182.

QUESTIONNAIRE

(To be filled by lady doctors only)

Do you find your work environment stressful?

If you do, please answer the following questions:

Area: _____   Respondent No._____

A) BIO DATA

   1. Name:_____

   2. Father's Name:_____

   3. Address:_____

   4. Age:_____

   5. Qualification:_____

   6. Current Status of Job:_____

B) OCCUPATIONAL HISTORY

1) Do you think the workload is too much for you?
   (Y___N___)

2) Do you think you work more than the required hours?
   (Y___N___)

3) Do you find your patients non cooperative?
   (Y___N___)

4) Do you experience peer pressure within profession or withotherprofessions?
   (Y___N___)

5) Do you find your training a long and tedious job?
(Y___N___)

6) Are you troubled with social expectations and obligations?
(Y___N___)

7) Do you have a hostile job environment around you?
(Y___N___)

8) Do you more often criticize yourself?
(Y___N___)

9) Are you suffering from the 'burnt out phenomenon' (a triad of emotional exhaustion, depersonalization and low productivity/achievements)?
(Y___N___)

10) Does the burden of administration solely rest on you?

(Y___N___)

11) Do you feel you have lack of time, recognition and autonomy?

(Y___N___)

12) Is the staff around you supporting enough?

(Y___N___)

13) Do you find your salary low?

(Y___N___)

14) Do you have dependent family members like mother, father, sister etc.?

(Y___N___)

15) Do you have disabled and sick family members at home?

(Y___N___)

16) Are you afraid of the risk factors of diseases at current working place?

(Y___N___)

17) Are you fed up of studies and exams?

(Y___N___)

18) Do you have the fear of insecurity?

(Y___N___)

C) FOR MARRIED WOMEN

1) Do you think you have been overloaded by playing multiple roles in society?
   (Y___N___)
2) Do you have a major work family conflict?
   (Y___N___)

3) Has your husband's behavior in any aspect affected you psychologically?

(Y___N___)

4) Are you satisfied with your household tasks, housekeeping and bringing up of your children?

(Y___N___)